Cosmic
Flow

Cosmic Flow

A Creative Guide to Harnessing the Rhythm of the Moon

★

Nikki Strange

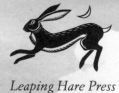

Leaping Hare Press

First published in the UK and North America in 2020 by

Leaping Hare Press

An imprint of The Quarto Group
The Old Brewery, 6 Blundell Street
London N7 9BH, United Kingdom
T (0)20 7700 6700
www.QuartoKnows.com

British Library Cataloguing-in-Publication Data
A catalogue record for this book is available from the British Library

ISBN: 978-0-7112-5348-3

This book was conceived, designed and produced by

Leaping Hare Press

58 West Street, Brighton BN1 2RA, United Kingdom
Publisher David Breuer
Art Director James Lawrence
Editorial Director Tom Kitch
Commissioning Editor Monica Perdoni
Project Editor Elizabeth Clinton
Design Manager Anna Stevens
Designer Hanri van Wyk
Publishing Assistant Chloe Murphy

Printed in China

10 9 8 7 6 5 4 3 2 1

Contents

My Story

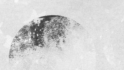

Few things have helped me more than discovering the power of the moon. For eight years, I've run a design and accessories business; as many self-employed folks can testify, it can be a lonely life. You have to make all your own decisions; there's no boss or colleagues there to validate your success or to give you approval, which can be a challenge in an increasingly digital age that moves so fast. It's easy to feel disconnected and like you'll never keep up.

When I began to slow down, though, I realized that, for all my worry and stress, I knew what to do. I might feel like I didn't, but when I could think things through and tune into my intuition, the answers were there. Why else, really, had I created my business in the first place? I had a passion for beauty and for finding a higher purpose; I just needed to learn to trust it. This was what inspired me to explore the lunar cycle. I wanted to understand how to harness this magical source of the divine feminine; to tap into my instincts with confidence, to feel comforted and cared for in moments of fear and doubt. I wanted to learn to use this energy, not just with work, but as an ongoing self-discovery project in every aspect of my life.

My love of this energy shows itself through all my design work and paintings, as well as the product range I evolved to help others self-care through planning and journaling. I hope this book helps you enjoy the transformation that can unfold when you work with the moon.

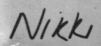

Working With The Moon

Embracing lunar energy means embracing cyclical living. Everything has a beginning, middle and end, and you can thrive in the delightful certainty that whatever happens, the cycle will begin anew next month, providing you with a new opportunity for discovery and beginnings.

In this book, you'll be learning to get in sync with the energies of the moon during its eight different phases. You'll start the journey at the new moon, where you'll learn to manifest and set your intentions; you'll then work to cultivate your energy so you can start putting your desires into action as the moon waxes. When the moon is full, you'll reflect on your journey so far, then adapt your energy during the waning phase to let go and release blocks, embracing a sense of gratitude for where you are and giving help and service to others. By creating this rhythm and flow in your life, you can conserve your energy, using it wisely.

This process helps you adapt better to change, be it seasonal, personal, or in your relationships with the people and world around you. It can also help you see the lessons that reside in everything: the beautiful parts of human experience as well as the painful; the pleasantly surprising, the unexpectedly hard, and the miracles. Working in this way helps you remember that nothing is fixed. Whatever is happening, look to the moon: it'll shine down the reminder that it's all just another phase.

How To Use This Book

Before you start your way through the exercises in this book, print out a chart of the moon phases. (You can find these online in your correct time zone.) That way, you'll always know where you are in the cycle and how many days you can expect each phase to last.

Each of the eight chapters in this book represents a distinct part of the moon's cycle, so begin with Chapter 1, on the day of the new moon. I'm writing this book in the Northern hemisphere; if you're reading it in the Southern hemisphere, the moon phases will appear reversed in the sky, but the meanings and stages will remain the same.

There are exercises in every chapter for that particular stage of the cycle; you can do as few or as many as you like. Do what intuitively feels right for you, and bear in mind that some phases last longer than others.

Once you've worked through the book for your first lunar cycle, you can start again at the beginning. You may have manifested your intentions and be in search of new ones; you may still be working on them and want to adapt a bit, or you may have decided they weren't what you really wanted and feel the need to set something quite different. Listen to your own feelings, and let them be your guide.

The Sun & Moon

From where we stand on earth, the moon seems to change shape. The view from space, however, is rather different.

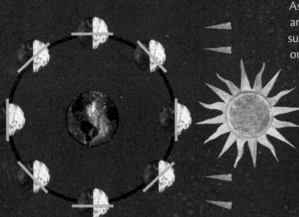

As the moon revolves around the earth, the sun always illuminates one half of it. You can see how this changes our view from season to season and phase to phase.

Yin & Yang Energy

Throughout the ages, the sun and moon's energies have been seen as opposites, with the sun often being considered masculine/yang energy and the moon feminine/yin. Both these energies rest within us too; they reveal themselves in our outward presentation, our conscious feelings and our subconscious emotions.

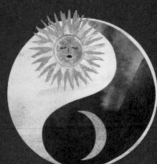

Sun	Moon
Yang	Yin
Masculine	Feminine
Radiant	Tranquil
Glowing	Emotional
Vigorous	Shadowed
Confident	Receptive
Passionate	Reflective

Sun Energy

Write words inside the sun that describe the personality
you shine outwards to other people.

Curious

Kind

Giggly

Giving

Eager

Stubborn

Dreamy

Hopeful

Compassionate

Gentle

SOft

sensitive

Intuitive

Emotional

Self-Aware

Moon Energy

Write within the moon words that describe your quieter self,
the private feelings you hide.

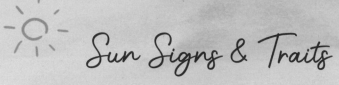

Sun Signs & Traits

The earth orbits the sun every 365 days, which means it sits in each of the 12 zodiac signs for approximately 30 days before moving on. The cycle starts in Aries and finishes in Pisces; this is known as the 'astrological year'. How do the traits of your sun sign below relate to what you wrote for your sun energy activity on page 11?

Aries
THE RAM
21 March - 19 April
Independent, strong-willed, playful

Taurus
THE BULL
20 April - 20 May
Level-headed, realistic, materialistic, dependable

Gemini
THE TWINS
21 May - 20 June
Dreamer, intelligent, charismatic

Cancer
THE CRAB
21 June - 22 July
Emotional, sensitive, creative

Leo
THE LION
23 July- 22 August
Extrovert, fiercely loyal, artistic

Virgo
THE VIRGIN
23 August - 22 September
Efficient, organized, witty

Libra
SCALES
23 September - 22 October
Balanced, diplomatic, generous

Scorpio
THE SCORPION
23 October - 21 November
Protective, powerful, sensual

Sagittarius
THE CENTAUR
22 November - 21 December
Optimistic, adventurous, philosophical

Capricorn
THE GOAT
22 December - 19 January
Practical, logical, hard working

Aquarius
THE WATER BEARER
20 January - 18 February
Humanitarian, kind-hearted, inventive

Pisces
THE FISH
19 February - 20 March
Highly sensitive, empathetic, compassionate

Moon Signs & Needs

The moon orbits the earth every 27.5 days, and moves through each zodiac sign every two and a half days. This is why you need to know your time and place of birth to find your moon sign: if you do, you can use an online generator. How do the needs of your moon sign below relate to what you wrote for the moon energy activity on page 11?

♈ Aries
Creativity, thinking for yourself

♉ Taurus
Aesthetics and nice possessions; financial security

♊ Gemini
Mental and social stimulation

♋ Cancer
Nurturing, family (biological or chosen), being by water

♌ Leo
Self-expression, attention

♍ Virgo
Healthy and productive routines

♎ Libra
Security through partnerships; tact and kindness

♏ Scorpio
Passion, devotion and commitment

♐ Sagittarius
Challenges and room to explore

♑ Capricorn
Tangible goals leading to a sense of achievement; emotional self-protection

♒ Aquarius
Feeling part of a greater community

♓ Pisces
Transcendence, self-expression through creativity

Four Elements

Each of the zodiac signs are housed into four elements: air, fire, water and earth. These groups make up our universe; each has its own distinct energy that, when combined together, create versatility and balance.

What are the element groups for your sun and moon signs? Write below some of the attributes you see in yourself, both for the signs and their element(s). Is the energy different for your sun and moon signs?

Air
Gemini
Libra
Aquarius

Intellect
Communication open minded
Free-spirited thinking

Dreamy/understanding
Hope Wishful Intelligent
Whimsical intel

Fire
Aries
Leo
Sagittarius

Action
Passion
Drive

_____
_____

Earth
Taurus
Virgo
Capricorn

Materialism
Stability
Practicality

MARS × SATURN
_____

Water
Cancer
Scorpio
Pisces

Emotion
Sensuality
Creativity

_____
_____

Your Two Sides

Taking what you know of yourself, and looking at the energy of your sun and moon sign and element group(s), use the space below to draw the following. On the moon side, draw what brings you comfort and feelings of calm, home and belonging; on the sun side, draw what makes you feel passionate, energetic and radiant. You can draw objects, places, people, memories or whatever you like.

SUN - Libra 24.96° 5th
MOON - Gemini

Sun side   Moon side

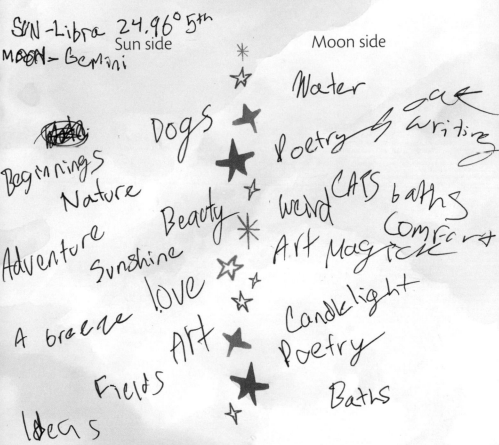

Water

Dogs

Beginnings

Nature

Poetry & writing

weird CATS baths

Art Magick Comfort

Adventure

Beauty

Sunshine

A breeze Love

Art

Candlelight

Poetry

Fields

Baths

Ideas

As you work through this book, use these as a visual reference when you need inspiration, or a reminder of what makes you feel supported and happy.

The Lunar Cycle

These are the eight stages the moon goes through during the lunar cycle. This 'lunation' takes 29.5 days, slightly longer than the moon's orbit around the Earth, as it includes the time it takes to go from one new moon back to the next.

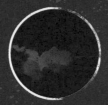

1 ★ New Moon

The moon is dark in the sky, and it's a time of beginnings – an opportunity to connect with where you are right now, and meditate on your desires, gifts and passions, and what you want to share with the world. Setting your intentions can create a conscious connection with what you want in life.

2 ★ Waxing Crescent

When there's a slight curve in the sky, the moon is emerging from darkness and starting to grow (wax). This is a time to explore those thoughts and desires you mapped out. It is fun and challenging to work on aligning your energy and beliefs to the intentions you've set. Trust yourself: you are finding your unique magic.

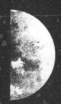

3 ★ First Quarter

The moon appears as a stark semicircle in the sky. Midway between new and full moon, it's time to start putting your intentions into action. Be willing to disrupt patterns and adjust your routines; you are tapping into your higher purpose and pushing towards what you wish.

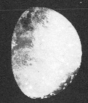

4 ★ Waxing Gibbous

As the moon grows ever rounder in the sky, so does your newly cultivated energy. Now that you are actively working towards your intentions, it's also a time to stay motivated. Trust your process, looking for signs and miracles that offer reassurance of the universe's support.

Get familiar with each stage, noting how the moon gradually waxes (that is, gets bigger) until it reaches fullness, and then gradually wanes back to darkness. The time of waxing and waning stages varies from five to eight days, month to month.

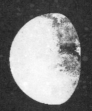

5 ★ Full Moon

The moon is swollen with light, and it's a day to reflect on your journey so far. The full moon can heighten emotions, so it's a time to stay connected with the present moment, immersing yourself in nature and ritual so you don't get overwhelmed.

6 ★ Waning Gibbous

The moon begins to diminish in size, and you can ask yourself where you are right now. It's time to shift your energy from manifestation to gratitude, passing on positive feeling to others.

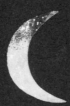

7 ★ Third Quarter

The moon appears again as a semicircle, but this time reversed. At this time you can go inwards to connect with your shadow side, opening up to your less comfortable feelings. Embrace the art of self-love, showing yourself compassion and being ready to let resentments go.

8 ★ Waning Crescent

The moon dwindles to a small sickle, going back into darkness so the cycle can start once again. Now is the moment to restore your energy; prioritize rest, comfort and nourishment. Let your soul wind down, preparing to harness the power of the next new moon when it appears again.

Moon Gazing

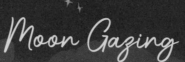

Using the chart on pages 16–17 as a guide, go out this evening and observe the moon. Draw it below and work out what phase it's in; it may be slightly bigger or smaller than the pictures on our chart but you should be able to get a good approximation. If you can't see it, there's a good chance it's new, but you can check what phase it's in online if you're not sure.

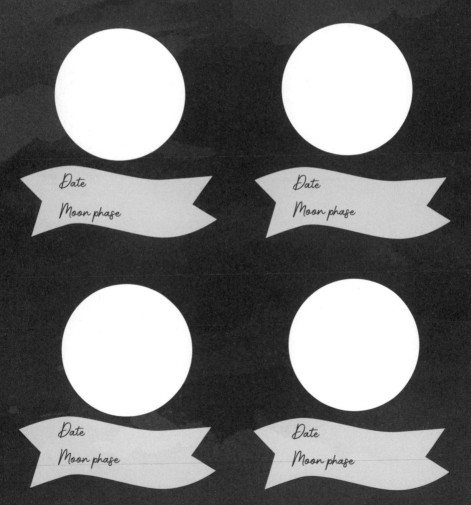

Date

Moon phase

Date

Moon phase

Date

Moon phase

Date

Moon phase

Stepping out of doors to do this will help you get in the habit of looking up at the moon, which is so much better than just looking online when it comes to connecting to the moon's energy. Once you become familiar, you'll start to know where the moon is in her cycle instinctively, so build a diary below.

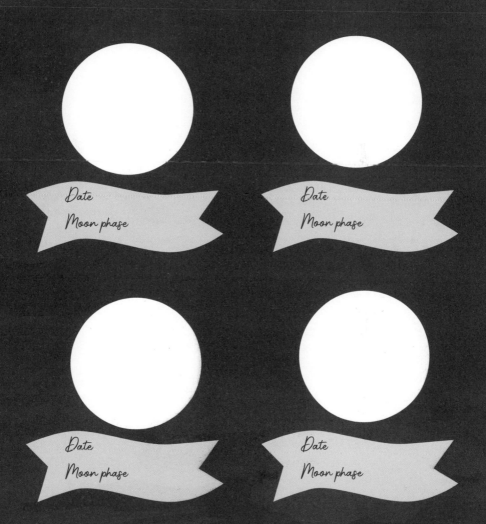

Date

Moon phase

Date

Moon phase

Date

Moon phase

Date

Moon phase

The Triple Goddess

The moon is about the divine feminine energy, connecting you to your emotional, intuitive side. You can do this no matter whether your gender is female, male, or non-binary; these are aspects everybody has. The triple goddess symbol helps us understand the idea a little better, through the archetypes of maiden, mother and crone.

Waxing Crescent
THE MAIDEN

The waxing crescent moon is associated with the maiden, an icon of exploration into the unknown, taking action with courage and optimism.

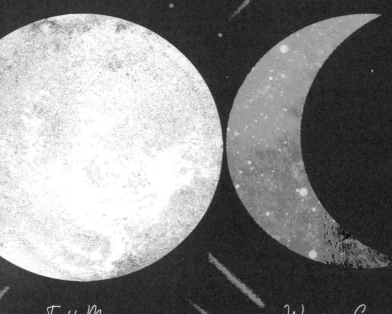

Full Moon
THE MOTHER

The full moon is associated with the mother. The focus here is on compassion and self-care; that maternal energy that embraces all. She also embodies fertility and a productive spirit; you may see your intentions beginning to take form.

Waning Crescent
THE CRONE

The crone contains ancient wisdom. She's no old hag, as patriarchal fables would have us believe; instead, she is wise, strong and enduring. Experience has weathered her and taught her to survive trauma, follow intuition and know when to rest.

Create An Altar

Your altar is your very own, a space to bring about personal change and create individual rituals. For this reason, I'm not going to throw a 'must have' list at you; instead, this is a series of suggestions you can adapt according to your own emotional needs and practical capacity. Working around the elements of fire, earth, water and air can be an inspiring way to start; you can make things big or small, have one candle or many, be lavish or modest. It's all up to you.

Items for your ritual:

Lavender

CANDLES ○

CRYSTALS ○

INCENSE ○

SMUDGE STICKS ○

SENTIMENTAL OBJECTS ○

ORACLE OR TAROT CARDS ○

HERBS ○

FLOWERS ○

INTENTION LIST OR AFFIRMATIONS ○

Use the space below to design the altar you'll set up in your own home.

★ What size works best?

★ What do you want it to call in?

★ What makes it intrinsically 'you'?

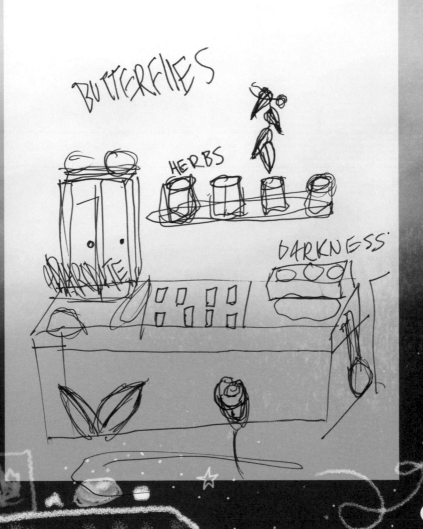

Chapter 1

NEW MOON

Set Your Intentions

When the
moon is hidden in the sky,
it's a time of new beginnings.
Get ready to call in change and
make a conscious connection with
what you want in life.

New Moon Energy

During its (just under) 28-day orbit around the earth, the moon passes through all 12 zodiac signs, spending about two and a half days in each. This means that with an understanding of each zodiac sign, we can work with the moon's energy to gain guidance throughout the month. In particular, it's helpful to know which sign the moon is in when it's new: that way, we can bring our new-moon ritual into focus on that sign's unique aspects. (To find out which sign it's aligned with, compare the date of the new moon to the date of the sun signs on page 12.) Listed below are the key zodiac energies, to help you start every month on the right path.

Aries is associated with taking action. It leads the start of the astrological year and sparks initiative. Set intentions that focus on courage and new beginnings.

Taurus is associated with the material, things we can touch and feel. Set intentions that focus on finances, prosperity and treating yourself.

Gemini is ruled by Mercury, the planet of communication. Set intentions that focus on building relationships and personal expansion.

Cancer is ruled by the moon, making it an emotional sign with a focus on family, and on things that make you feel secure. Set intentions that focus on home and loved ones.

Leo is an eccentric sign, with traits of self-expression and creativity. Set intentions that focus on playfulness and exploration.

Virgo is associated with stability through organization and planning. Set intentions that focus on wellness and cultivating beneficial habits.

Solar Eclipses

A solar eclipse takes place when the sun and moon are in alignment, meaning that from where we stand, the sun is blocked, either in part or in full, by the new moon. This celestial event is a catalyst for change and rebirth, bringing even more potency to that new-beginnings energy. Keep an eye out for them and think big with your intentions.

Libra is concerned with harmony. Set intentions that focus on balance and on connecting with others.

Scorpio is a sensual sign with strong emotional associations, helping us explore the full spectrum of our psyche. Set intentions that focus on feelings and personal goals.

Sagittarius is associated with higher wisdom and discovery. Set intentions that focus on learning and adventure.

Capricorn is about sustainable achievements and practicality. Set intentions that focus on strategy and long-term achievement.

Aquarius is associated with forward thinking and pioneering change. Set intentions that focus on community and generous thinking.

Pisces evokes the mystical realms and thinking beyond the physical. Set intentions that focus on intuition and spirituality.

New Moon Ritual

When the moon is new, it's time to reconnect with yourself: dig deep into your own desires and reflect on how you want your life to change. By making time for a ritual now, you can plant the seeds of what you want to blossom in your future.

This ritual is flexible, and can be done alone, or with friends, in a quiet space where you won't be disturbed. Doing the ritual with friends can be a great way to add momentum to your intentions collectively with the unity of your energies combined.

The aids below aren't mandatory; they're suggestions to help you experience a sensory exploration. This can give you deeper clarity, while also calling up memories. Such things add a sense of specialness to your ritual, giving you that giddy feeling of excitement in your belly.

For myself, I like to set up an altar with candles, a crystal that resonates with the energies I want to call in, and some visual aids that reflect what I want to manifest. If you don't have these to hand, don't worry. What you need most is to turn off your phone, shut out distractions, and get quiet so that you can engage with the place where the magic happens: your mind.

You will need

★ **An altar space setup (see page 22)**
★ **Music**
★ **Comfy cushion to sit on**
★ **Candles or incense**

Take a deep breath and note how you feel right now. Identify any sensations in your body, such as aches or tight spots, and the thoughts currently floating through your mind.

How I feel before the ritual:

— Longing... For love? For more?
— Lonely? — Am I to blame
— Neck/shoulder/back pain

If you've decided to use candles or incense, light them. Set your music playing. Listen to your breath; try to breathe slowly and calmly, as settling your body helps settle your mind. If your attention wanders, listen to the sounds around you.

After a few minutes, you hopefully should start to feel relaxed. Now, think about your intentions – that is, what you want to call into your life. Do you have any desires, or inklings of them? If so, write them down. The changes might be monumental or subtle. Don't judge yourself; just be open to what you want.

Inklings and desires that I'm feeling:

Write down your intentions. Pick between one and ten, as many or as few as feel right for your situation. This is a list you can refer back to throughout the lunar cycle.

My intentions:

Slowly, one by one, go through the intentions you set. Allow each to come into your mind's eye; visualize it playing out as a story. Let yourself get fully into it, feeling the emotions as if the events were really happening right now.

How does it make you feel to watch the tale unfold? Make note of colours, tastes, smells, sounds, or revelations that became apparent during the visualisation, really communicate what you felt onto paper.

What I experienced:

Once you've worked through your intentions, sit in stillness and let gratitude wash over you like a wave. Imagine your intentions have come into fruition. You have now planted the seeds of what you want to accomplish: enjoy the sense of security that brings you.

I ALIGN MY

energy

WITH THE

changes

I WANT TO

call in

Visualize Your Future

With one of your intentions in your mind's eye, draw it below. Embrace your playful side; you can use crayons, collage, whatever makes it vivid to you.

It's In Your Hands

On the spiral line inside the crystal ball, write a narrative of your intention from the page opposite. Describe the scene or the object and how it's part of your life.

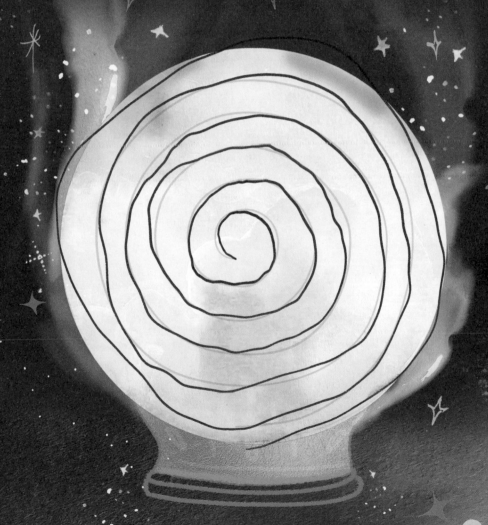

The Night Sky

Either going outside or looking from your window, take time to gaze into the dark. What can you see there? Clouds, comets, planets? The subtle colours of an electric-shaded city sky? Can you see any of the 12 constellations pictured here? Using pencils or pens, draw what you see; include any trees, buildings or obstructions to give a sense of where you are.

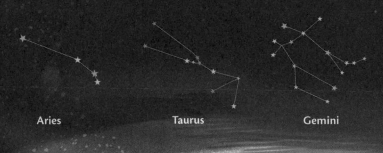

Aries   Taurus   Gemini

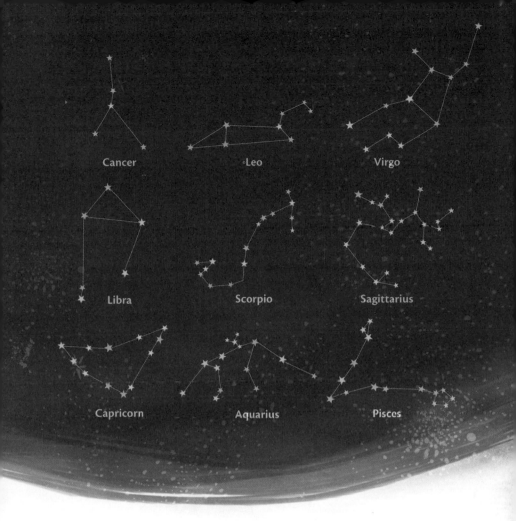

Cancer

Leo

Virgo

Libra

Scorpio

Sagittarius

Capricorn

Aquarius

Pisces

My Happy Place

Imagine yourself a month from now, and a year from now. Draw yourself in your ideal happy place, identifying the short- and long-term goals you have set. What would surround you? Who would be keeping you company? This is what you're trying to manifest.

Vizualize being here, and remember, this is an imaginative place you can visit any time.

1 month from now

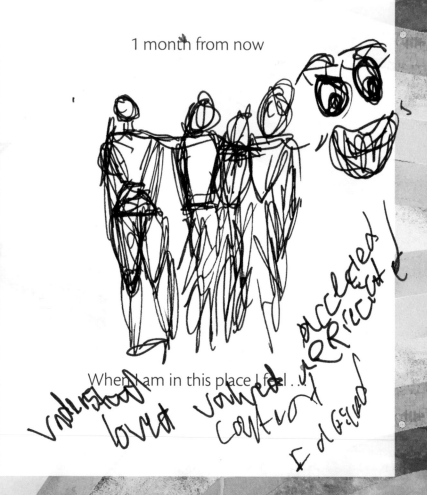

When I am in this place I feel . . .

1 year from now

Traveling

France 1.

Greece

Amsterdam 3.

Ireland

Spain 2.

When I am in this place I feel ...

fulfilled   curious
            inspired

Kali Energy

Kali is a Hindu goddess associated with death and destruction leading to rebirth. This makes her a perfect goddess to look for within ourselves as the lunar cycle begins. She is about destroy limiting beliefs, and looking for that crack of light within the dark.

She is often depicted as black or blue, her neck adorned with a chain of decapitated heads, tongue unfurled, and each of her multiple hands holding a sword. As such, she is seen as a representation of *shakti*, a Sanskrit word evoking universal cosmic energy, associated with the divine feminine, powerful but not to be feared. When the sky is dark and the moon new, we can call on Kali's energy to destroy our self-limiting beliefs, imagining her swords slashing away the ties of bad habits and self-sabotage. Stagnant energy can keep us feeling stuck; Kali's potency clears that all away.

Take a moment to go inwards. How do you view yourself? When you consider who you are at the moment, what words come to mind? Write them down quickly, without self-censoring, then look at what's there. Are there any beliefs holding you back, patterns that need disrupting to create a dramatic transformation?

victim? Survivor a warrior
not breable independent
lonely mis understood

40

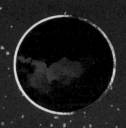

Colour in your vision of Kali

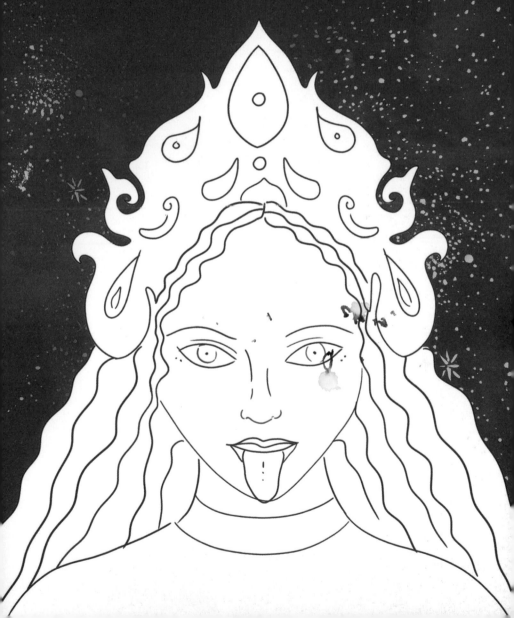

Chanting

Your throat chakra can get clogged with negative energy, making it harder for you to speak your truth; singing and chanting are great ways to clear it. Mantras are an ancient way of doing this, elevating the spirit through the repetition (out loud or silently) of a word, phrase or sound, often in Sanskrit. Below are two such sacred sounds, which have been used in Kundalini yoga for centuries. Kundalini yoga works on the principle that energy runs up from the base of your spine through your chakras, and that, with the right exercises, you can unleash it. They're a great thing to use during new moon, when you want to refresh your thought patterns.

Har
The Creative Infinity

This mantra helps unlock abundance and prosperity. Don't be misled by the spelling: it's actually pronounced 'hu-duh', your tongue bouncing hard off the roof of your mouth.

With your eyes closed, chant 'HAR' in your mind over and over, for about three minutes. Once you've become comfortable with the sound, chant it out loud for three minutes. Try and pulse your navel when you breathe, aligning your breath to the rhythm, and then, once you're settled into that, bring your focus to your third eye chakra. This is the space between your brows, associated with insight.

If you can sustain it longer, try for 11 minutes, but be advised, that can be challenging!

Note how you feel afterwards below:

Satnam
Truth, Identity

This mantra is a Kundalini yoga staple, and used during
many exercises to help focus the mind.

When chanting, try to visualize this energy rising up through
your root chakra (that's the lowest one, around your bottom three
vertebrae and between your legs), rising up through your body,
energizing you all the way to the crown of your head. Sat Nam is a great
mantra for accessing your true nature, helping you come back to yourself
when you've been too much in your own head.

Chant 'SAT NAM' inside your mind for about three minutes. Time it so you
have 'SAT' on your in-breath and 'NAM' on the out-breath, again using your
navel as an anchor for your focus.

Then bring your attention to your third eye chakra and imagine your energy
flowing up through your body, root to crown. Chant the mantra out loud
for three minutes, or as long as you can manage.

Note how you feel afterwards below:

Shake It Out

Below, write a list of songs that always get you excited to be up and moving.

My playlist:

Put your playlist on and dance, letting the music travel through you. Dance around; be silly and expressive. Wiggle, jiggle, shake those fingers and toes. Feel the energy moving from your root chakra up through your body. What stirs inside you?

As soon as you finish your dance, before your heart stops racing, sit down and quickly write how you feel. Are there any particular inspirations or joys you want to record?

How I feel after letting my body dance:

Do you have any new desires or
insights that could stimulate new intentions?

Did any particular lyrics make you
feel uplifted or motivated?

I Am

How we talk to ourselves affects what we believe, and that can change the energy we bring into our lives. To help manifest your intentions, it's great to write how you'd feel if they'd already come to pass. This lets you experience new, positive energy, seeing past the experience of just being stuck.

On the page opposite, write out one or two intentions, not as wishes, but as part of your reality. For instance:

'I AM living compassionately,'
or
'I AM a brilliant artist.'

Do these expressions make you feel doubtful or scared? Write a mantra to support the aspiration, for instance:

'I AM patient and kind to myself on this journey ahead.'

Make them look fun and representative of your personality; write neat or wonky, graphic or playful, using colour to enjoy the new mantras you are creating.

Once complete, sit in stillness and let the sense of what you have written fill your body. Invoke this new, bold energy: it's what will power new thoughts, and the new actions that will follow them. In this way, you're getting ready for the next stages of the waxing moon.

I AM

I AM

I AM

Chapter 2

WAXING CRESCENT MOON

Settle into your intentions

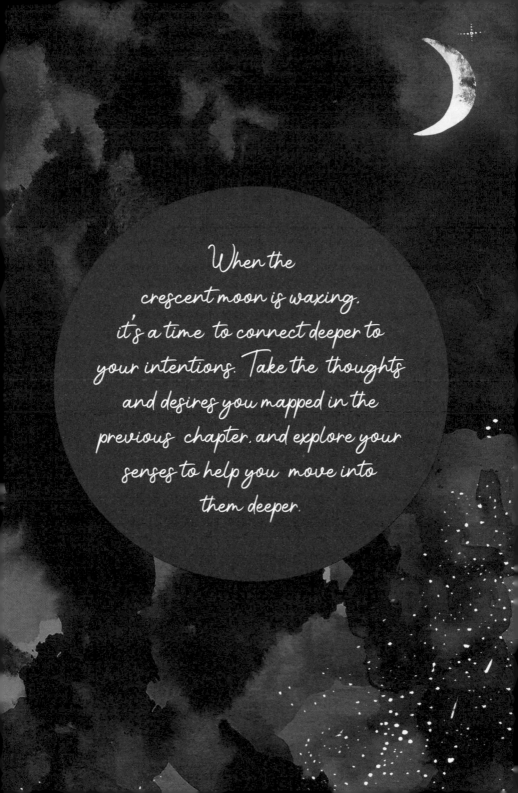

When the
crescent moon is waxing,
it's a time to connect deeper to
your intentions. Take the thoughts
and desires you mapped in the
previous chapter, and explore your
senses to help you move into
them deeper.

Maiden Goddess

With the slim curve of a crescent growing fuller in the sky, the moon is waxing. At this time, we look to the 'maiden' archetype from the trinity of goddesses (see page 20). Artemis is the Greek goddess to invoke here: she is fearless, youthful and free-spirited. Often depicted hunting in the woods, armed with a bow and arrow, a deer by her side, she is a huntress and protector of nature. By embodying some of her enchanting spark, we can connect to our adventurous, uncompromising ambitions. Sit in stillness, and think how you'd like to call this up in yourself.

Above, list ways to be more courageous in your daily life, achieve your aspirations, and face the world boldly.

Artemis is the virgin huntress, goddess of wildlife and protector of animals. Draw a natural setting of flowers, trees and beasts. Think, as you do, how to connect more to nature and embody that nurturing energy.

Planting The Seed

When you put an intention out into the universe, it's like planting a seed deep in the earth. You nurture it patiently and allow it to grow, confident it will one day bloom. Think like a gardener: it's the whole process of growth, not just the end result, that is important.

Type of plant ....

Intention it represents ....

....

Date planted ....

There's a belief that the gravitation of the moon
pulls water higher in the soil during the waxing
stage of the lunar cycle, swelling seeds. As the nights also
become brighter, it's a good time for plant growth. Pick something
you'd like to plant – indoors or out, depending on your resources –
and associate it with a long-term intention that may need time to
develop. It will act as a gentle reminder of the power of patience.

Over the coming months, return to these pages to draw and document the
growth of your plant. Has your intention progressed too? There's space here
to do this for a second plant too.

Type of plant ....

Intention it represents ....

....

Date planted ....

Wish You Were Here

POSTCARD

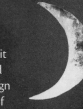

Writing as if from the future can really add some energy when it comes to acting on your intentions. This is a particularly good exercise when the waxing crescent moon is in Gemini, as this sign is all about clarity and communication. Write your current self a postcard from future you, describing the life you have, what you see, where you are, and how you feel.

You can even use the stamp to draw a little self-portrait, and the address section for where you'd like to be.

Inspirational Resources

Use the space on these pages to record art and media that will aid your growth and help you fulfil your intentions. These may include resources for spiritual development, planning, finance, travel – whatever will help you learn, excel and motivate yourself. Do this regularly to keep from stagnating and stay inspired.

Books
Title/author/how it will help

Podcasts
Title/creator/how it will help

Workshops or courses
Course name/location/how it will help

Films and documentaries
Title/director/how it will help

Websites or social media accounts
Site/handle/host/how it will help

My Inner Child

Being busy, we often neglect our playful sides. Looking back at what you loved as a child is a great way to reconnect with this: when we were children, we did what we did for the sheer delight of it. Allow yourself some nostalgia: it'll enrich your life by bringing back forgotten joys, and help you understand and refine your new-moon intentions.

Don't focus on what you were 'good at'. Think about what you were drawn to, or passionate about.

Things I loved as a child:

How I felt when I was doing these activities:

Can you see any connections between what you wrote here and what brings your 'moon side' comfort (see page 15)?

Read over what you've written. Does it stir an impulse to bring more of these feelings back into your life?

Try and make some time to do one of these activities, or else the adult equivalent. For instance, if you liked playing with clay, you could try a pottery class.

Below, document what your playtime reveals. It might help you with your intentions, either for this lunar cycle or one in the future.

Crystal Tuning

Did you use crystals in your new moon ritual? If so, pick one out: it should be one you felt drawn to, and small enough to carry with you. Write below some words that bring you comfort and guidance; let them flow freely. They don't have to make logical sense. They just need to be words of unconditional love.

Now, sit and recite them while holding your crystal. By charging it with this energy, it will give you extra support. Keep it close to help spur you on and give you that bit of extra courage, a talisman you can hold on difficult days.

Words of encouragement:

I TURN

inward

TO FEEL

supported

AND GUIDED

Affirmations

Now is a time to really believe what you're calling into your life can come to pass. Daily affirmations can help here, as they reinforce positive beliefs and help to quiet any negative inner voices. It's a quick and easy way to realign your energy if you start feeling off track.

Begin by repeating the following affirmations five times in your mind, slowly, letting them sink in. Then say them five times aloud. It can feel silly at first, but it really does add potency.

**'I have enough time to get
done everything I need to do today.
I am able to take small breaks to relax,
which will help me stay
focused and calm'**

**'I will slow down today
and be patient with myself.
I will pay extra attention to
small joys to keep myself present in my life'**

**'Today I will be helpful
and of service to others,
remind myself of the
bigger picture and
pass on this kind energy'**

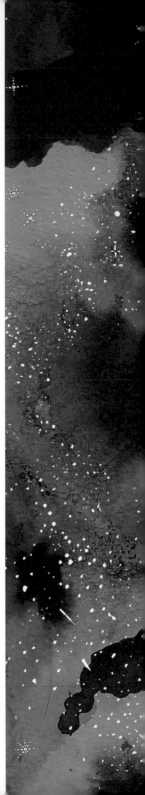

Now tailor the affirmations to your needs or create your own. Write them down below. Try and repeat these daily or when you can for a few minutes to make a shift in your thought patterns.

 Each lunar cycle, come back to this page and write any changes you've experienced. This will let you see the magic happening.

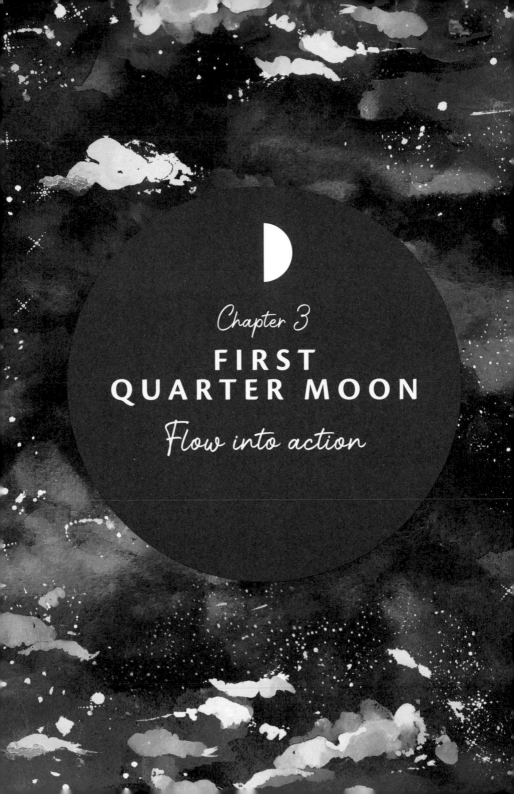

Chapter 3

FIRST
QUARTER MOON

Flow into action

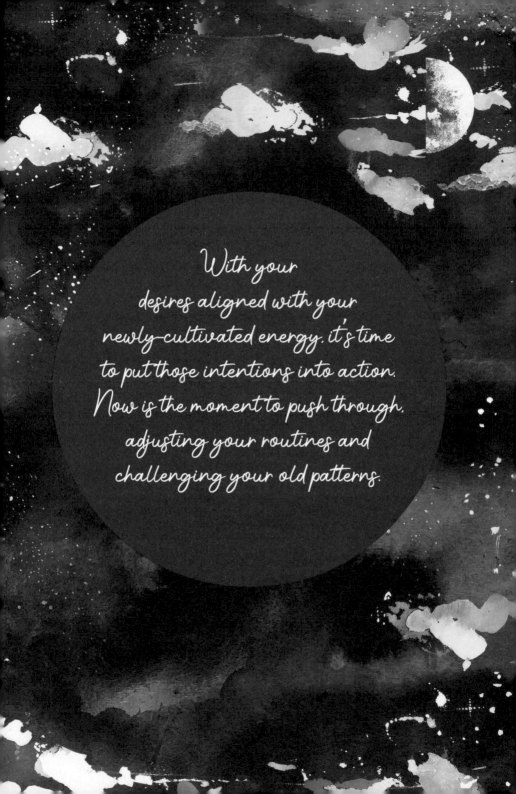

With your
desires aligned with your
newly-cultivated energy, it's time
to put those intentions into action.
Now is the moment to push through,
adjusting your routines and
challenging your old patterns.

Stepping Stones

When you have multiple intentions, it can be a bit overwhelming: where do you start? Look at your list from page 31. Some will be short-term goals and some will take longer to accomplish; use the steps below to work out which are which.

Phrase or word to summarize intention

Define the time frame: short-term or long-term

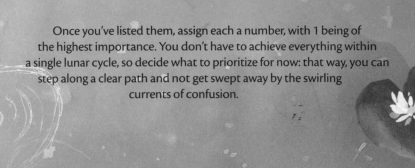

Once you've listed them, assign each a number, with 1 being of the highest importance. You don't have to achieve everything within a single lunar cycle, so decide what to prioritize for now: that way, you can step along a clear path and not get swept away by the swirling currents of confusion.

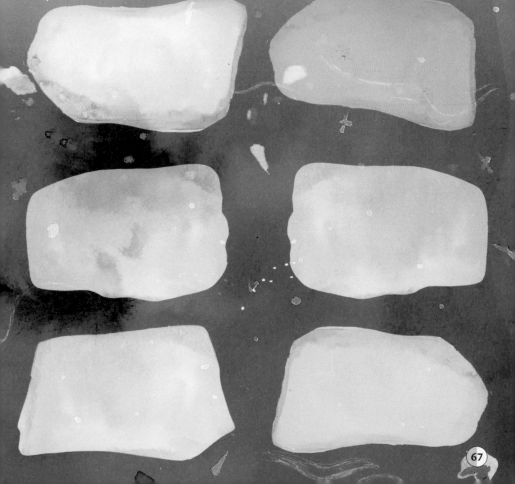

Purpose
(be specific)

How it will make
you feel

The
Butterfly Effect

Focus on one of your intentions, just one for now. How will it serve you, your loved ones? Might it even touch your wider community? (Though it might not, which is fine.) Write down what you envision. This exploration can show you how important it is that your intention comes to pass. Spreading love and support adds a value to our lives no material pleasures can touch; you may even feel inspired to re-evaluate your intention or recommit to it as you explore the prospect.

How it will serve me and improve the quality of my life:

How it will affect my close friends and family:

How it will affect my wider community:

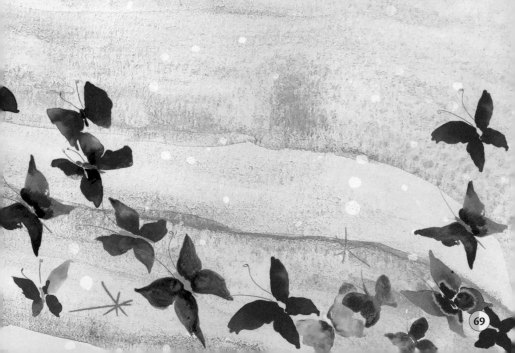

Dear Me . . .

Look at your list of intentions; you can pick out a few, or tackle them all. Close your eyes, and imagine them as a fully-fledged reality; picture them as clearly as possible. Now write yourself a letter to remind yourself why you want these things to happen. Be unapologetic and passionate. When you feel the need to keep yourself motivated in future, you can come back here and reread it, so write with kindness and positivity. This is a place to give yourself some pep.

Dear me,

_____

_____

_____

_____

_____

_____

_____

_____

_____

_____

_____

_____

Flow into action

Using this flow chart, record the progress you're making as you put one of your chosen intentions to work. Write down all the actions you can take, then come back and tick them off as you accomplish them.

Remember that sometimes things don't happen as quickly as we want. Take that as an opportunity to re-evaluate if you're completely ready for the intention to manifest; if progress is slower than you hoped, don't fret, as it may just be the universe giving you more time to prepare. Use these notes to remind yourself of all you've done, and be aware that we can't control everything. The more you let go of that expectation, the more open you will be, and the better able to spot unexpected magic and opportunities showing up around you.

Intention

Positive actions I've taken

◯ _____ ◯
_____ ◯ _____ ◯
_____ ◯ _____ ◯
_____ ◯ _____ ◯

Concerns
or issues

Signs it's
coming to fruition

Actions
I can still take

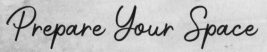

Prepare Your Space

Visualize a place you use often, be it at home, work or outside. What changes would you make to this space to help bring your intentions to life? Maybe you're ready to make a big transformation, creating the environment of your wildest dreams, or maybe you just want to tidy and organize to make more room for productivity and creativity. Draw a plan below, adding annotations on where you'll store things, or patterns and textures you might add. Invite change into your life.

I PUT

into action

THE CHANGE

I want

TO SEE

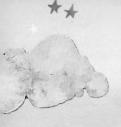

Clear Your Headspace

Our minds are filled with constant chatter, making it hard to see what's really going on in there. Writing down how you feel can help separate out the important parts, letting you see them clearly before you. Are there any negative thoughts or emotions, such as fears or anxieties, sabotaging your actions right now? What's the evidence for them? Write them out: if they're practical obstacles, you can plan for them, and if they're irrational fears, you can let them go.

Negative thoughts	Evidence for negative thoughts
Negative emotions	Evidence for negative emotions

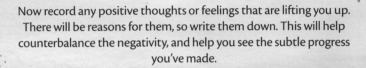

Now record any positive thoughts or feelings that are lifting you up.
There will be reasons for them, so write them down. This will help
counterbalance the negativity, and help you see the subtle progress
you've made.

Positive thoughts

Reasons for positive
thoughts

Positive emotions

Reasons for positive
emotions

Chapter 4

WAXING GIBBOUS MOON

Explore & refine your desires

When the
moon waxes gibbous, that's
a time to stay motivated: even
when things seem ordinary, trust in the
process, looking for the tiny miracles
that show you are supported. In this
phase, you can adjust your
intentions so they always
reflect where you are.

Positive Energy

With our daily routines and busy schedules, it's easy to fall into sensible habits and end up feeling guilty if we have any fun. Your life needs positivity and silliness, though. Use the prompts here to explore the little things that make you feel good and lift your spirits. Adding more pleasure to your day actually helps you keep committed to your new-moon wishes. We all know resolutions can get broken when we lose motivation, so during the waxing gibbous stage, a light heart that embraces joyful moments will support you keeping faith with your intentions.

Things that relax me and get me offline

Things that make me feel free

Things that make me laugh uncontrollably

Songs that instantly make me feel good

Activities
I can fit into
10-minute breaks
throughout the
day

Ways to get
out into nature

Write below any ideas on how you can implement
these activities into your daily life.

Escape Your Comfort Zone

Taking risks is scary, particularly when our minds keep over-thinking and coming up with false reasons to be afraid. Fear is a natural emotion and exists to keep us safe, but it's important to remember that you truly do have the power to take risks and push your capabilities. Check out the mountain opposite: write at the base the beliefs you feel are holding you back, and then list some ways you might power through those limits. At the top, write the things that scare you in a good way: the heights you want to reach.

Uncomfortable
but learning

Ways to push through

My limiting beliefs

Ripple Effect

We can't always predict all the outcomes when we set an intention, but that can be a good thing. Have you noticed any positive changes that have resulted indirectly from your new mindset? Shifts can occur that add a richness to your life you didn't expect.

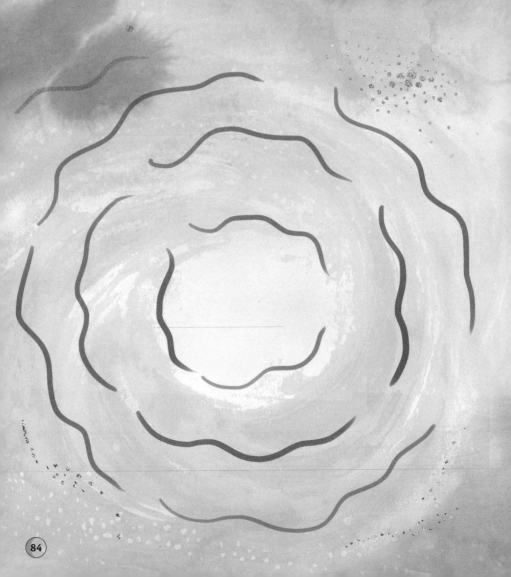

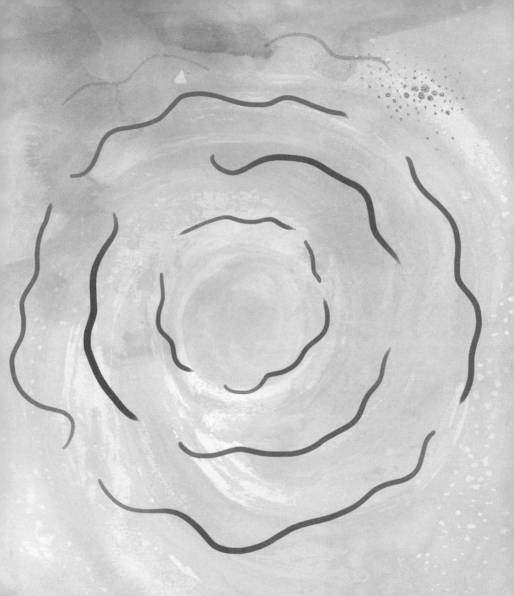

If nothing like that has happened, it's a good time to have a think about the real purpose behind your intentions. Do they still feel aligned with what's right for you? Often we 'want' things because we fear we are lacking something in our lives, or we believe once we achieve the end goal we will be happy. Here's an opportunity to check in and ask: are my intentions for the good of myself and others? Do they encourage learning and self-development? Do they still ring true to me?

Weighing Up

Sit holding one of your intentions in mind. Play it out: if it came into fruition, what are the positives and negatives that could result? By being practical, you can get a clearer vision of how your plans and dreams will affect your life. That way, you can test whether they are well balanced to serve your higher self, and also decide whether you need to change anything in your life to make room for them.

Pros
Good, positive things that will happen if my intentions come into being

Cons
Issues that may occur if my intentions come into being

Control

Now you've begun acting on your intentions, think about what might be affecting your power to manifest them. Some of those things will be outside of your control, so write them down. Acknowledging that reality helps take the pressure off you. Some things will be within your control, however, so write those down too. In this way, you'll have a comforting, written reminder that you are doing all you can.

Things I can control

Things I can't control

Observe Your Habits

Pick out two days within the gibbous moon period for these pages. Make a note of what you did, both interesting events and mundane ones. Be specific: you want an accurate record. When you're done, take an honest look at how you spend your time, and see if there are any habits of self-sabotage you'd be better without.

Day One

6am

7am

8am

9am

10am

11am

12pm

1pm

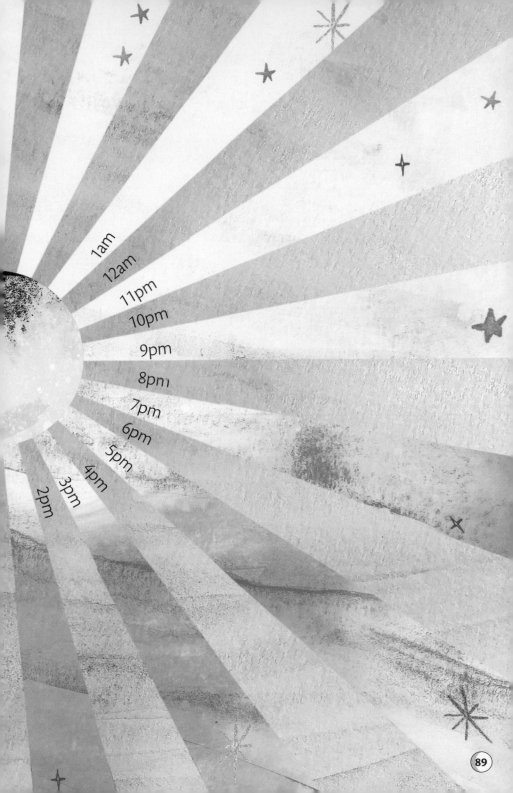

1am
12am
11pm
10pm
9pm
8pm
7pm
6pm
5pm
4pm
3pm
2pm

Day Two

Reflect on your day and use the space below to record what you've discovered. Note any reasons you might be undermining yourself.

6am

7am

8am

9am

10am

11am

12pm

1pm

1am

12am

11pm

10pm

9pm

8pm

7pm

6pm

5pm

4pm

3pm

2pm

Words With Feeling

It can be hard to stay motivated when you set an intention and it doesn't seem to be coming through. To help you through those moments of frustration, use this page to record resonant quotes, be they from poetry, prose, speeches, interviews or whatever else makes you feel supported. They don't have to be over-the-top motivational proverbs; just sentiments that embrace the human experience as you understand it.

Trust In The Process

Go outside and sit in sight of a tree. We often don't pay the magnificent living forms around us enough attention: trees adapt from bloom through decline to rest every season, a reminder we need this cycle in our own lives. Draw the tree before you, colour, bark, scale and all (you can add other objects to show the size), noting where it is in its cycle. Remind yourself that you are connected to this living form and its ancient wisdom. This perspective can help to quiet our incessant internal monologue.

Take a look at your new-moon intentions. Did stepping out for some fresh air change how you saw them? Write about how you could refine them from this new perspective.

Unexpected Miracles

Think of a time when, unexpectedly, something remarkable happened.
Sometimes letting down our guard makes space for a magical shift;
it doesn't have to be big, but it can still feel like a miracle. Think
of a time when this happened to you, and use the space
opposite to narrate the event, describing how you
felt, both before and after it happened. Use this
as a reminder to trust that the universe is
working with you, and that struggle
is not a sign of doom, but a
chance to learn.

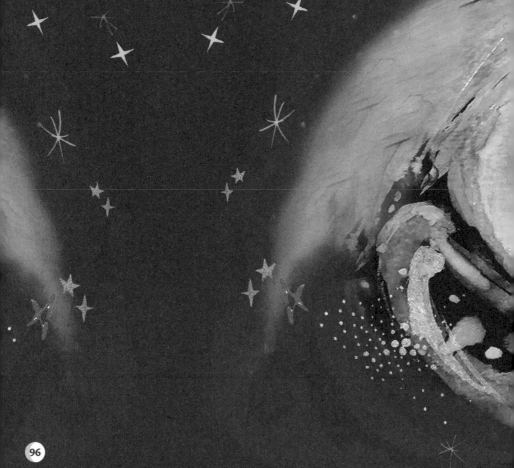

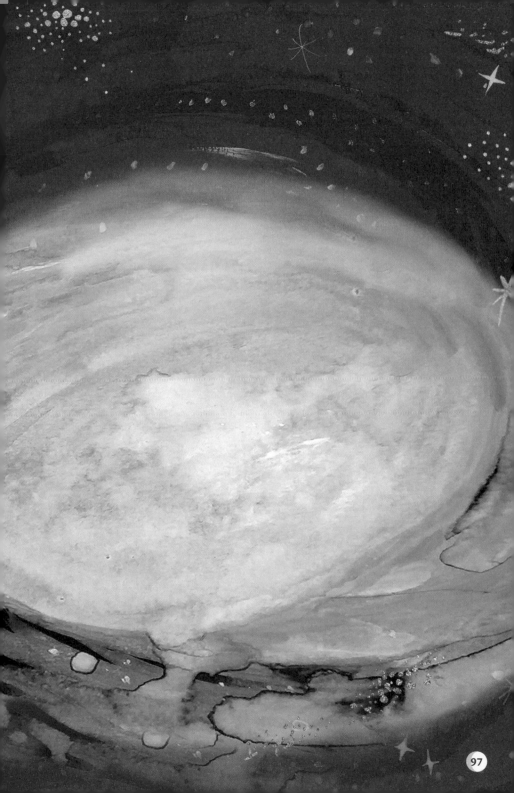

Signs From The Universe

A sign, or synchronicity, happens when something seems beyond a coincidence. It holds a personal resonance with you, as if the universe is giving you a gentle nudge, or a mystical wink. These can be anything, from a vision in a dream, recurring events, seeing lucky numbers or hearing the right lyrics on the radio, to an unexpected gift or some good news that opens up new opportunities to follow your intentions. Here, write, draw, collage or doodle anything that makes you feel like magic is at work.

I PAY

attention

TO THE

signs

THAT ARE

guiding me

Your Support Network

During this waxing phase of the moon, it's important to trust that, no matter what intentions you set, whatever is happening at this very moment is what should be. If the results aren't obvious, that can be unnerving, so draw below the people who make you feel supported and held in tough times.

Next to each person, write how they do this, or the feeling you get from their energy. Remember: that feeling is available to you at all times.

You can take this further by confiding in someone you trust. Share with them your intentions and the progress you've made so far. If they give you any wise words, note them below: they may provide you with a fresh approach. Include anything they say that you disagree with, too; in another lunar cycle, you may find their comments resonate more.

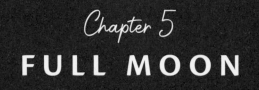

Chapter 5

FULL MOON

*Acknowledge your
intentions & release
negativity*

The full moon amplifies emotions. To avoid being overwhelmed, connect to the present moment and experience your true nature, letting yourself be nurtured by the positive, maternal energy of this phase.

Full Moon Energy

Each month, the full moon will be in a different zodiac sign, and focusing on the energy of that sign for your full moon ritual is a good way to look at your challenges through a new perspective. The mathematics of working out which sign it's in is slightly complicated, so the simplest solution is to check online.

♈ Aries

Focus on your confidence and your independent spirit. Face challenges as a bold pioneer.

♉ Taurus

Get connected with your body, your appetites, your sense of deservedness. Be hungry for positive change.

♊ Gemini

Connect with others: new thoughts and fresh approaches may be just what you need. Communicate; knock ideas around; share inspirations.

♋ Cancer

Use this energy to empower your creativity. With courage, your emotions can lift you to new heights.

♌ Leo

Express yourself. We're all unique individuals; embrace that, accepting what comforts and encourages you as valid and rightful.

♍ Virgo

Get yourself organized. It's a time for clarity, clearing away mess and building a stable foundation from which to act.

Lunar Eclipse

When the full moon passes directly behind the Earth,
our planet casts a shadow that seems to darken it.
Be alert to this astrological event that signifies endings
or major changes.

Libra

Keep yourself balanced.
Be in harmony with
others, and treat your
own emotions with
patience; that way, you're
poised to respond to any
positive change with
discernment.

Scorpio

Feel the full force
of your desires and
sensuality. You have
the power to transform;
let your emotions be
the fire that creates
the alchemy.

Sagittarius

Use this energy to
draw you towards new
discoveries. Be honest
and open; it's a time
to let your natural
wisdom lead you along
the right path.

Capricorn

Release resistance.
You are secure; think
about pragmatic routes
to your goals.

Aquarius

Look to the future.
Every good thing moves
you forward, so be
grateful and loving as
you anticipate your
next step.

Pisces

Use this energy to
transcend. Seek
out music, poetry,
whatever gets you most
in touch with the
mystical.

Full Moon Ritual

Without judging yourself, reflect on your intentions: what's coming to the surface, and what isn't? The full moon is a time to let yourself be raw, to uncover your deepest emotions and let them speak to you.

The ritual on the following pages can serve as a foundation, but adapt it freely and use intuition to make it truly your own; adding objects and themes of your choosing can help it reflect the essence of your life.

You will need

- ★ Sage, tied in a bundle, for smudging, and something to light it
- ★ Music that touches your emotions
- ★ Your list of intentions
- ★ A pen or pencil
- ★ An altar space of your choosing (see page 22)
- ★ Crystals or objects that connect with your intentions or with things you'd like to let go

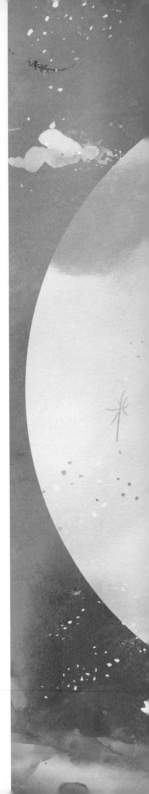

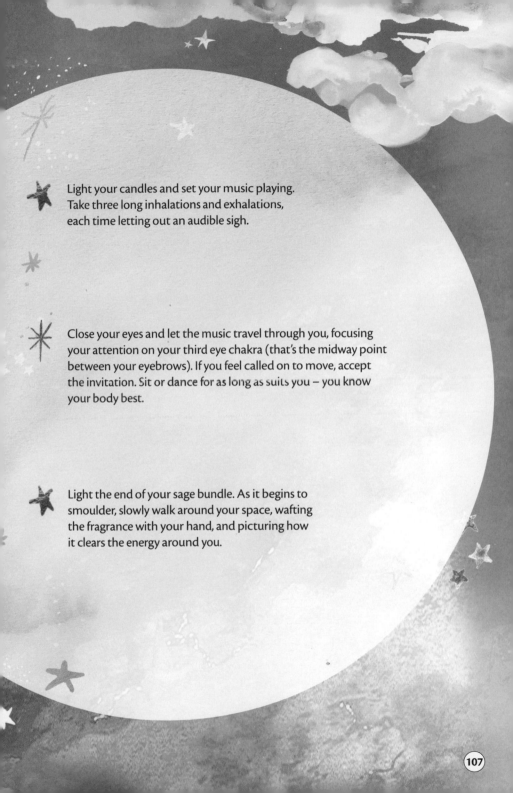

Light your candles and set your music playing. Take three long inhalations and exhalations, each time letting out an audible sigh.

Close your eyes and let the music travel through you, focusing your attention on your third eye chakra (that's the midway point between your eyebrows). If you feel called on to move, accept the invitation. Sit or dance for as long as suits you – you know your body best.

Light the end of your sage bundle. As it begins to smoulder, slowly walk around your space, wafting the fragrance with your hand, and picturing how it clears the energy around you.

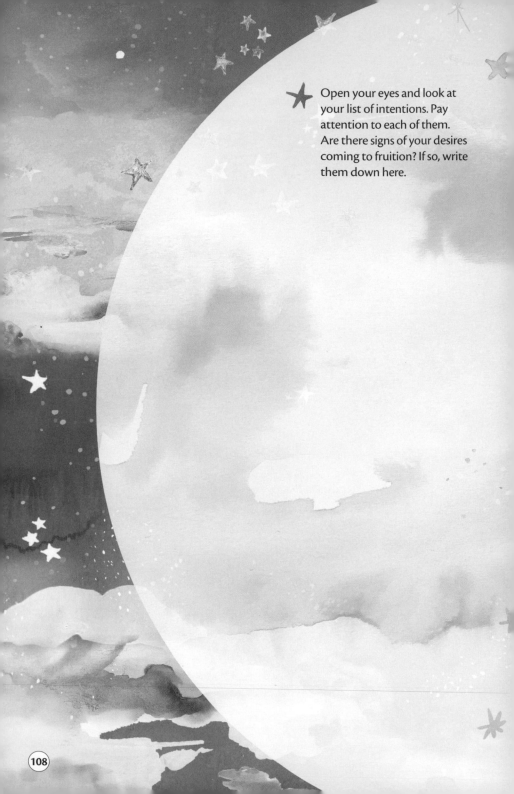

Open your eyes and look at your list of intentions. Pay attention to each of them. Are there signs of your desires coming to fruition? If so, write them down here.

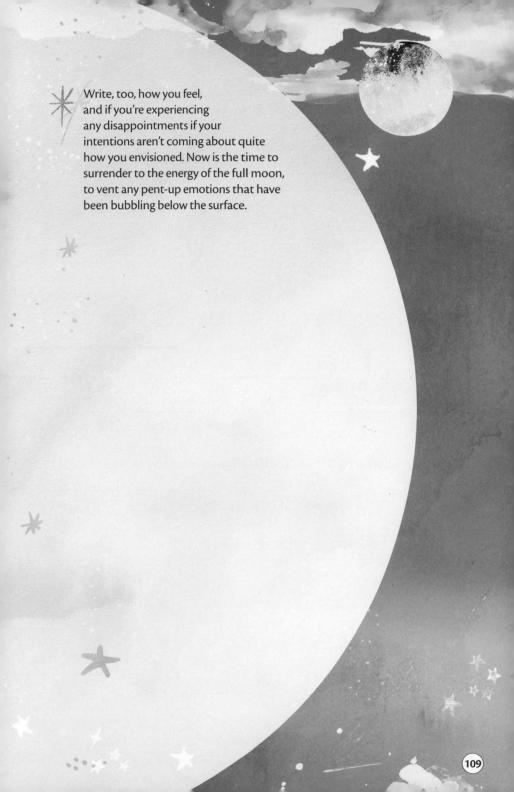

Write, too, how you feel, and if you're experiencing any disappointments if your intentions aren't coming about quite how you envisioned. Now is the time to surrender to the energy of the full moon, to vent any pent-up emotions that have been bubbling below the surface.

Let any strong feelings make themselves known. Don't fight them; just record how you feel, and allow yourself to forgive any negativity or frustration.

Emotional

Sensitive   Overflowing

Insecure

Defensive

 Tense

Pent-up

Pain +
Stress

Bring the meditation to an end. Use this space to record your reflections; they can help give direction for the next phases of the lunar cycle.

I MAKE

time

TO EXPLORE

how I feel

AT THIS

very moment

Chakra Scan

In Sanskrit, the word *chakra* means 'wheel'; we can picture chakras as spiralling fields of energy throughout the body, and they need to be kept in balance. There are seven main ones, which you'll see below, and each has its own colour, forming a rainbow.

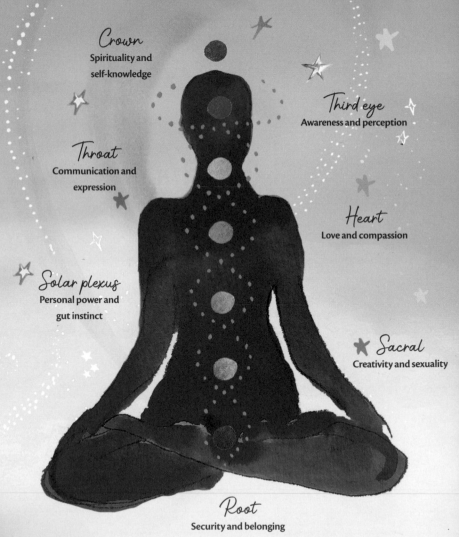

Crown
Spirituality and
self-knowledge

Third eye
Awareness and perception

Throat
Communication and
expression

Heart
Love and compassion

Solar plexus
Personal power and
gut instinct

Sacral
Creativity and sexuality

Root
Security and belonging

A simple chakra scan meditation can get you present in your body, and help you notice if you're holding any tensions there. Close your eyes and lay your hands against your root chakra; envision the deep red that permeates it, and rest there for two minutes. On the chart below, write any sensations you find. Then repeat this with your other six chakras, picturing their unique colours, working up towards the crown.

Limited   Mild connection   Distrust skepticism

Purple?   Lowered   Open Receptive

Blocked / Barriers   Stuck   pushed down withheld

Bursting Decompart mental   Secure in myself   Recent impessing guarded   Recreation

Bright   Tight Hot Radiating

Knotted + Twisted   Pent ve   Tight Bursting Rigid

TENSE   GUARDED   Sinking Disempowered

Look at what you have written. Does anything suggest a chakra that's blocked or overstimulated?

Do the scan again, but this time send purifying energy to each chakra. Imagine the coloured light cleansing and restoring you.

Mother Goddess

The second aspect of the triple goddess archetype is the mother: she stands for fertility, compassionate love, and understanding. The Greek deity Selene is an incarnation of the full moon, depicted in a white chariot drawn by white horses. New ideas are born through her and she nurtures the vulnerable. During a full moon, when our emotions run high, connecting to her loving energy can provide comfort and reassurance.

Do you have any such worries you'd like healed? Write them here.

Worries of
- Safety - insecurities
- Money - Health
- Relationship

Meditate for a moment, connecting with her energy of unconditional love. Imagine golden light pouring down on you, through your crown chakra and filling up your every cell. Let this energy hold you, safe and comforted.

Draw yourself as the goddess Selene below. What would she say to console your anxieties? Write her answers down.

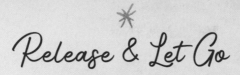

Release & Let Go

During a full moon, it's good to release any bottled-up emotions that could be holding you back. To do that, you need to be aware of them. To help find your obstacles and forgive yourself for any annoyance at them, write them below.

I release......*Co-Dependency*

and insecurities

I release..

....

I release..

....

I release..

....

I release..

....

Mandala

Mandala is a Sanskrit word for 'circle', and represents the nature of the cosmos with no beginning and no end. The full moon can make you feel over-emotional, so it's important to relax and unwind. Create your own mandala on the template below, adding different patterns and colours, as a peaceful meditation that helps keep you from over-thinking.

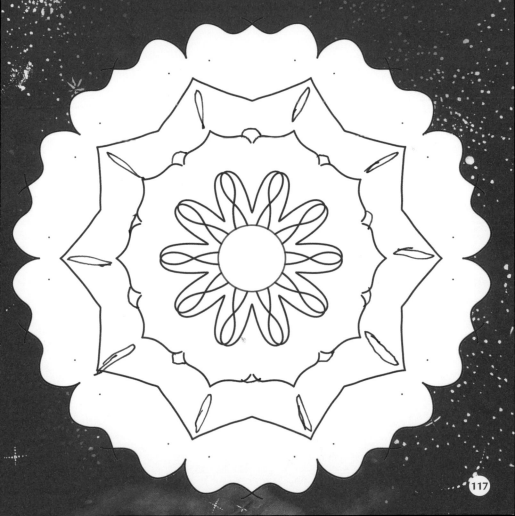

Moon Bathing

Go outside when the moon is bright and sit or stand barefoot on the grass. Imagine roots growing from your body, connecting you to the ground of Mother Earth and her energy.

Do any emotions arise? Record them below and make a note of what you can see, hear, smell and sense. If you're struggling for inspiration, focus on something you're usually too busy to notice: the sigh of the wind, or the intricacies of the bark on nearby trees.

Now that you've been energized by the moonlight, grab a pen and let it run freely on the page. Anything that comes to your mind, write it down, allow it to flow, even if it doesn't make much sense at this moment.

It's also a good time to cleanse your crystals. Put them in a bowl on your windowsill, or, weather permitting, outside. Let the energy of the full moon charge them.

Moon Gazing

Throughout history, the moon has fascinated us. Poets, writers and artists have been inspired by its romance, its loneliness, its wildness. Moon gazing entails sitting in its light and opening yourself up to its inspiration. Imagine its celestial energy beaming down upon you, as it has upon so many lives before yours.

Go outside and take a look at the moon. What do you notice? Is it bigger than on most nights? Shining with an unusual hue? Framed with clouds? This is a way to put our lives in perspective, letting our eyes rest upon a dazzling vision of something bigger than ourselves.

Below are some folkloric names of full moons that appear throughout the year.

JANUARY
Wolf Moon

FEBRUARY
Snow Moon

MARCH
Worm Moon

APRIL
Pink Moon

MAY
Flower Moon

JUNE
Strawberry Moon

My Moon Poem

Write a poem about the moon's beauty tonight. It can be short and sweet or long and descriptive. Don't worry about it being 'good'; this is a way to push out of your comfort zone and be present in the moment.

JULY
Buck Moon

AUGUST
Sturgeon Moon

SEPTEMBER
Harvest Moon

OCTOBER
Hunter's Moon

NOVEMBER
Beaver Moon

DECEMBER
Cold Moon

Get Creative

Put on some of your best-loved music. Then, using the space here, express yourself creatively. Make marks, shapes, lines, whatever flows from within you. Don't think, and don't try to create a polished end result, just let your inner child take over and have some fun.

Soaking Ritual

Make time for a soak in the bath as the moon glows. Get fancy with scented oils, petals and candles. Use an exfoliating scrub and picture it as scrubbing away old habits. After you're done, imagine any negative energy washing down the drain. This is an especially good ritual when the full moon is in Cancer, as that's a water sign and the moon is its great ruler.

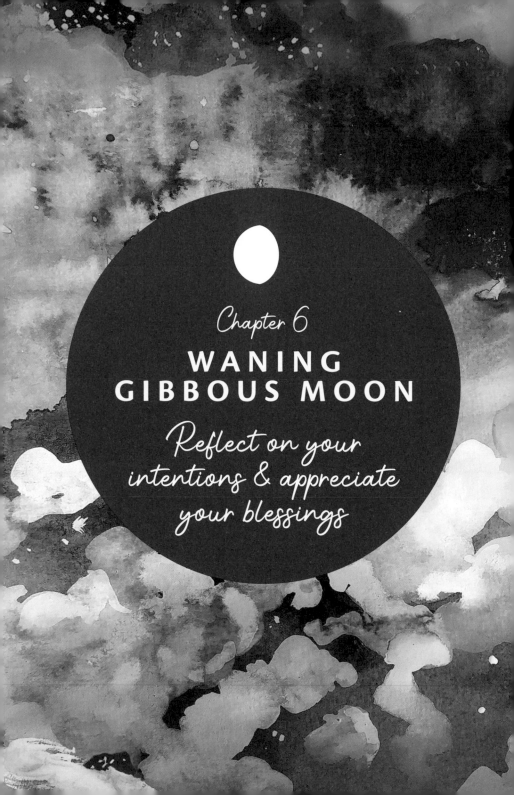

Chapter 6

WANING GIBBOUS MOON

Reflect on your intentions & appreciate your blessings

This phase asks
you to look at where you
are right now and appreciate
wherever that may be. Shift your
energy to a focus on gratitude rather
than manifestation. By being thankful,
you'll pass on this energy to others,
making time to connect and
serve with a purpose.

Reflect & Review

Take a snapshot of how you feel right now. Having passed the full moon, this is a perfect time to acknowledge, with thanks, what has come into being. Even the smallest wins are worth celebrating, so use the space below to record them. You want a true reflection, so feel free to record it if things aren't working out as you hoped too.

What has come into fruition

What hasn't that I was hoping for

- ★ †increased spirituality
- Meditation
- "Perfect setting"

- Rain + anxiety

What I should congratulate myself on

Doing My best
Giving Love

What changes I could make

Health changes

Self-discovery

Take a moment to write what you have learned during this lunar cycle about the process and how it affects you. Have you noticed changes, or found a new pace of life to help your self-development?

I've been focused on Selflove + co dependency. Limiting beliefs + an attempt to slow down

What have you learned about yourself? What wisdom would you share with others?

If you've been using this book for several lunar cycles, reflect on what you've written previously and how you've grown since then. This is a great way to really see how working with the moon has affected your life.

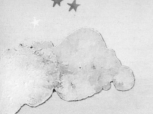

Say It Out Loud

Make a recording of you listing the things you're grateful for. (Your phone is probably the easiest way to do this.) Begin by announcing the date, so you can listen back and remember the context. Talk about your intentions and whether any of them show signs, however small, of coming to fruition; let yourself get excited. Being appreciative creates positive energy, which usually leads to you taking good actions that create more things to appreciate.

Below, write key themes from your recordings, including the date and time for easy reference.

Date & time   Key gratitude themes

Date & time   Key gratitude themes

Date & time   Key gratitude themes

Date & time   Key gratitude themes

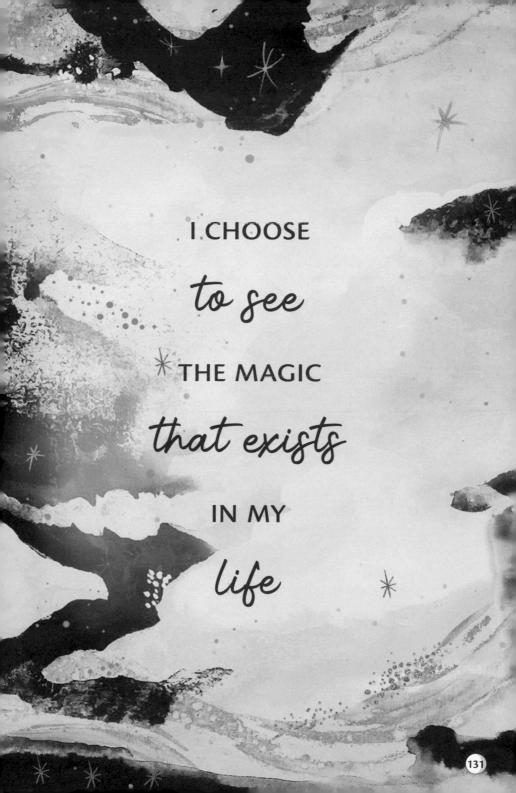

I CHOOSE

to see

THE MAGIC

that exists

IN MY

life

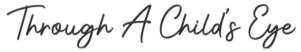

Through A Child's Eye

Picture yourself as a child again. What would little you be joyous about in your current life? Do you live with your friends? Do you wear wild, colourful clothing? Think about what impressed you as a child, maybe even dig out some pictures for prompts.

Write down or do a colourful drawing of what your small self would be most thrilled to know you have and do. And, in the spirit of your childhood self, don't worry about your drawing skills!

She'd be amazed IM OK, happy + trusting

Gratitude List

Below, write a short list of six things you're grateful for. It can include some of what you discovered in this chapter so far. You can also give gratitude to things yet to be called into your life.

Spend some time meditating on each one, letting that grateful energy rise through you. When you're done, write the list on a sticky note and put it up next to your mirror, or some other place you walk past every day.

Throughout the lunar cycle, look at those six things. Try saying them out loud as part of your morning ritual, or when you feel stressed or anxious; they'll create a positive shift in energy and make you feel better able to face the world.

★ 1. I am grateful for beauty and nature

★ 2.

★ 3.

★ 4.

★ 5.

★ 6.

Pass Those Feelings On

Now you've practised this warm loving energy, what could be more enriching than to pass it on to others? Explore how you can think bigger than yourself, connect, collaborate and help. It feels wonderful, and who knows, it might even bring some loving energy to you in return.

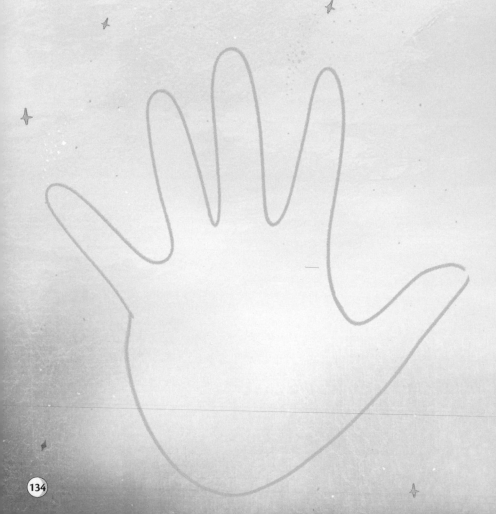

Above one of the hands below, write 'Community', and above the other, 'Family'. Imagine your energy flowing out through every fingertip.

On each finger and thumb, write down a blessing or energy you wish to pass on to that group. Then, around the outside of each finger, write down how you plan to pass it on.

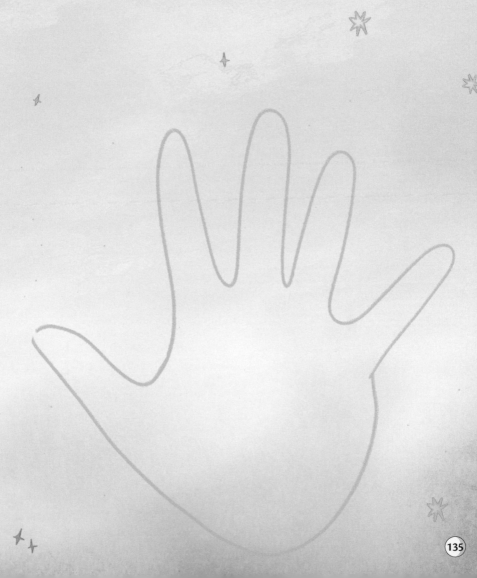

Small Acts Of Kindness

Think of five people in your life who matter to you, and whose lives you'd like to enrich.

Write some ideas of how you can do this. It could be a cute care package in the mail, a phone call asking how they are, a poem, a handmade gift or a home-baked treat. Whatever you choose to do, putting time, love and attention into something is the best gift you can give: it shows that you care, and gives you the chance to be creative as well. Include a planned date to give them this token, so you can space the acts out for a loving year.

Name

Why I've picked them

Act of kindness

Name

Why I've picked them

Act of kindness

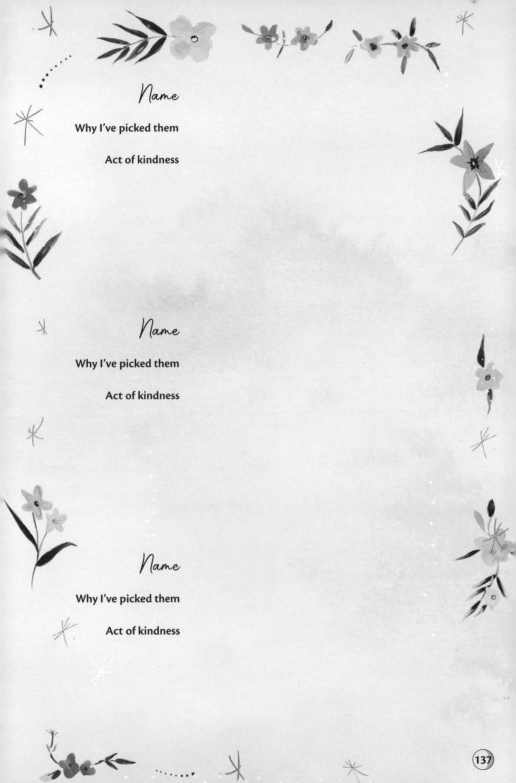

Name

Why I've picked them

Act of kindness

Name

Why I've picked them

Act of kindness

Name

Why I've picked them

Act of kindness

Pen A Letter

In this digital age, hand-written letters are becoming a lost art. Did you ever have a pen friend as a child? Do you remember the excitement of coming home to a letter on the table? Writing with a pen allows us to think differently: being more physical, we can write from the heart, feeling free to meander or get sentimental. So, take some time to write a letter to someone you haven't seen in a while. Reach out, letting your mind range freely. If you're stuck, try starting with a shared reminiscence, or include a quote you both like; whatever makes it personal between you and them.

Use the space below to brainstorm letter ideas.

Write a draft of the letter below, then take some nice paper and write a finished version, including sketches and drawings if you like.

Gratitude Graffiti

Use the space below to write a statement of the gratitude that fills you right now. Do bold, decorative text, as if you were tagging a wall. Then decorate the space around it; take your time, and enjoy your confident piece of art.

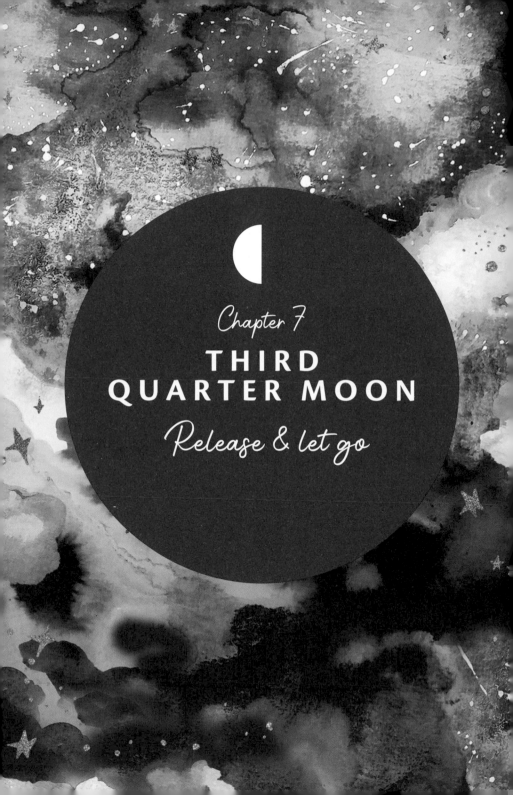

Chapter 7

THIRD QUARTER MOON

Release & let go

With the moon now at the
third quarter phase, go inwards to
connect with your shadow side. In this
chapter, you'll delve a little deeper into
those uncomfortable feelings, safely
exploring patterns and resentments
that need to be released.

Go Offline

Set aside a whole evening to go offline: put away all those devices. Instead, set a playlist running, made up of music that moves you, giving you a sense of catharsis and passion. Then, on some paper, write down five things you want to let go of. Be brutally honest: this list is for your eyes only and you'll destroy it later, so it's quite private. If you aren't ready to create a list yet, the activities later in the chapter will help you. When you're done, burn, bury or tear up the list, an act that closes the process and helps you shift the energy.

How did it feel to explore your feelings in a distraction-free setting? Write down any emotions and benefits you observe.

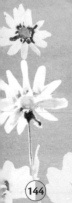

I ALLOW

myself

TO DIG

deeper into

MY EMOTIONS

Self-kindness

As the moon wanes, going into our shadow can help us explore the darker aspects of who we are, including feelings of shame and sadness. How have you acted during this lunar cycle? Below, list anything you did that left you feeling unsettled, annoyed, or upset, such as 'I felt bad I wasn't as supportive to my partner as I could have been.' Be honest.

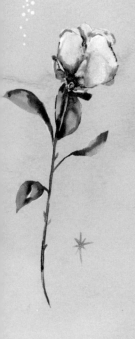

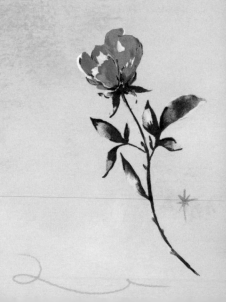

Now look at what you've written, and write a kind, empathic reply. Imagine you're talking to a friend. For instance, you could say, 'You were overwhelmed, and needed some time and space to recover.' The idea isn't to make excuses or blame others, but to show compassion and acknowledge that it's impossible to be perfect. In this way, you can start to be less hard on yourself.

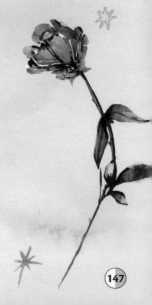

Clear The Air

Use the space below to write out any resentments or grudges you're holding either against a person or situation. Don't apologize: write down how they make you feel and how this has affected you. This is a space to release pent-up frustrations.

Now look over what you wrote. Is there a way to free up some of this stagnant energy? It's not a case of believing your feelings aren't valid, pretending that people didn't wrong you, or letting them take advantage again. Instead, it's about moving to a more healing mental space.

Hold the crystal you charged on page 119, or else some rose quartz, and feel that positive energy. Then write below how that makes you feel. Don't push yourself to achieve total forgiveness; just open up and embrace everything you feel.

Rise Above The Clouds

Is there anything blocking your progress with your intentions and life vision? Meditate on this for a while. Present day events can interfere, but so can childhood events and old thought patterns; think back to your earliest memories. If you find any fears, worries or limiting beliefs, write them on the clouds below.

Are there any realistic ways to remove these blocks? If it doesn't seem possible, that's also valid: write that down. Make a note of any repeating patterns or cycles you've spotted.

To help overcome these recurring thoughts, remind yourself of what you deserve in life, including the attainment of your goals.

I deserve . . .

I deserve . . .

I deserve . . .

Inner Monster

The ego can drive us to false beliefs about ourselves. These beliefs can leave us feeling that we're unworthy, not good enough, and prevent us from fulfilling our potential. We all have this 'monster' inside of us.

Draw your inner monster below. Once you've finished, write down all the things it tells you. Don't bottle them up inside: get them all out.

I am unlovable I'm clingy I am annoying Im worthless Im stupid, forgetful clumsy I dont deserve love I'm ugly

Seeing the things you tell yourself every day written down on paper can be quite shocking, and will hopefully reveal how irrational they can be. Once you spot how unnecessary this self-cruelty is, it can be easier to break the habit.

Inner Hero

Now you've got your demons out, use the space below to draw your inner hero or angel. Surround them with words of praise and support; write the things you'd tell a dear friend if you heard them disparage themselves the way the monster does you. This energy has power; make it your own.

I am deeply worthy of love
— Why?
I am allowed + encouraged to love
I hold value, I am wise +
Clever + smart. I am kind
Im beautiful. I am love,
I am loved, I am loving.

Lay your hand on your heart and feel its beat. Sitting in stillness, send yourself love. Imagine the energy of your inner hero sending you warmth; let it fill your body. What colour is this energy; what shape does it take? Add those to the picture too.

A Letter To Yourself

Write yourself a kind letter, praising the subtle things that make you your wonderful self. Be shameless: there are some great things about you. Never mind status or title. There must have been times when you helped, were kind, made someone laugh. When you feel good, you send this energy out to others.

Chapter 8

WANING
CRESCENT MOON

*Rest and prepare
to begin again*

The moon now
descends into darkness,
ready to begin the cycle afresh. In
this final chapter you'll be prioritizing
rest and exploring what gives you a
sense of comfort. In this way, you'll
restore your energy, preparing for
the manifesting energy of the
next new moon.

Moon-sign Comforts

Look to page 13 and think about what brings your particular moon sign comfort. Below, write what activities you could incorporate into your daily life to increase this cosy feeling. For instance, if you have a Pisces moon sign, you could read some poetry or fiction; if you are a Cancer, you could cook a wholesome meal. Try something different from your usual routine.

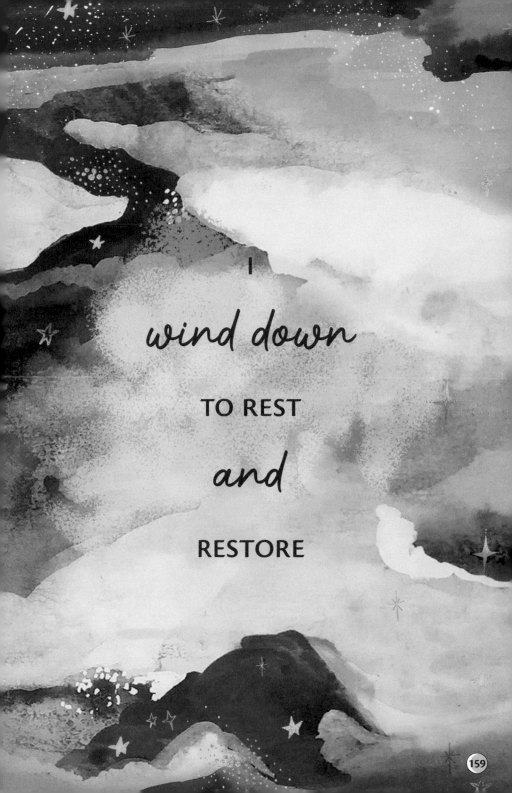

I

wind down

TO REST

and

RESTORE

Wind Down

During this phase, it's important to prioritize sleep so you conserve your energy for the next lunar cycle. Any bedtime ritual needs to be consistent, but at this time it needs to be particularly restful, so try the ritual below to help you wind down, release your thoughts and send out healing energy.

Healing sleep spell

You will need

* Dried lavender
* Calming essential oil (ylang ylang, chamomile, rose, geranium, or lavender)
* Small muslin or cotton draw-string bag
* Pen and small piece of paper

Ritual

 Fill your bag with the dried lavender, adding a drop or two of your chosen essential oil.

 On your scrap of paper, write down something you want to heal, either in yourself or someone else. Add it to the bag and draw the string closed.

 Sit and meditate, imagining this healing energy at work.

 Place the scented pouch under your pillow. You can refresh the scented oil whenever you need to.

Write down three things that you are grateful happened in your day, they could be things that were beautiful or made you smile. If nothing comes to mind, don't worry; just approach tomorrow alert to such possibilities, and write down three things that evening.

Morning Journal

When you wake in the morning, take advantage of that dozy, half-dreaming state and write down the first things that come to your mind. Don't worry if they make sense, or even if they're legible. Just use this space to put down whatever's in your mind when you first open your eyes, and stop as soon as you feel yourself becoming fully alert and aware. See this as a release at the very start of the day; let go of whatever has come up for you during the night.

Make Space

The waning crescent moon is a good time to clear out possessions and clutter, either by donating things or recycling them. Even tidying your living space and organizing your stuff helps realign your energy and brighten your mindset.

Use the space below to list what items you want to get rid of, and why. What energy will this remove or invite? Set yourself a time limit and, since energy dips are normal at this time of the lunar cycle, reach it by small steps.

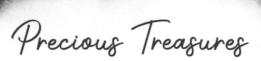

Precious Treasures

Draw here some of the things that are precious to you, holding great associations and memories. Next to each drawing, write why they matter to you so much. Looking at what we cherish can help us really value what we have, and also remind us that, rather than materialistic shopping, it's sentimental value that counts the most.

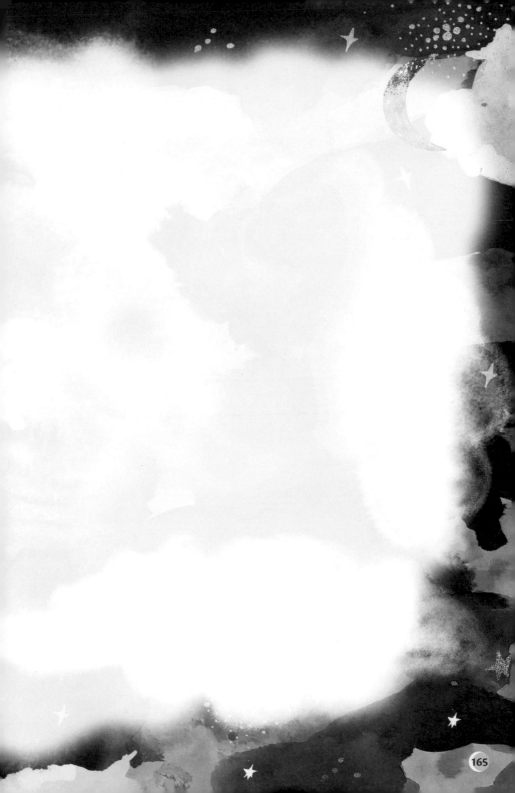

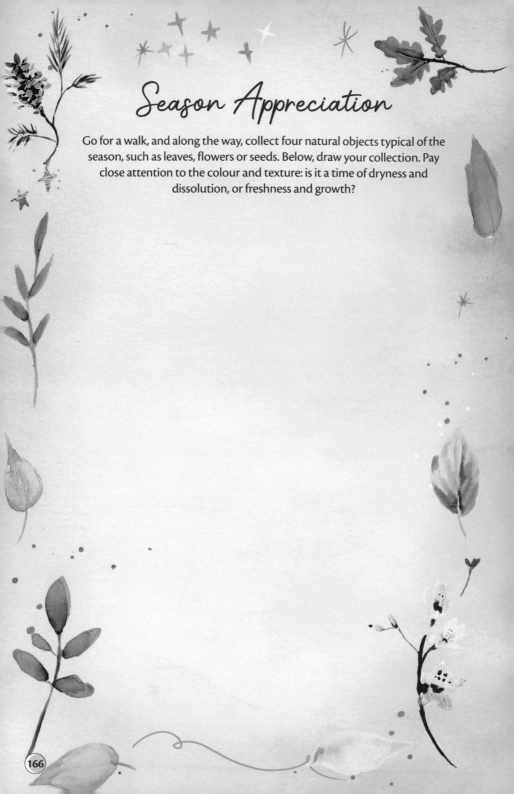

Season Appreciation

Go for a walk, and along the way, collect four natural objects typical of the season, such as leaves, flowers or seeds. Below, draw your collection. Pay close attention to the colour and texture: is it a time of dryness and dissolution, or freshness and growth?

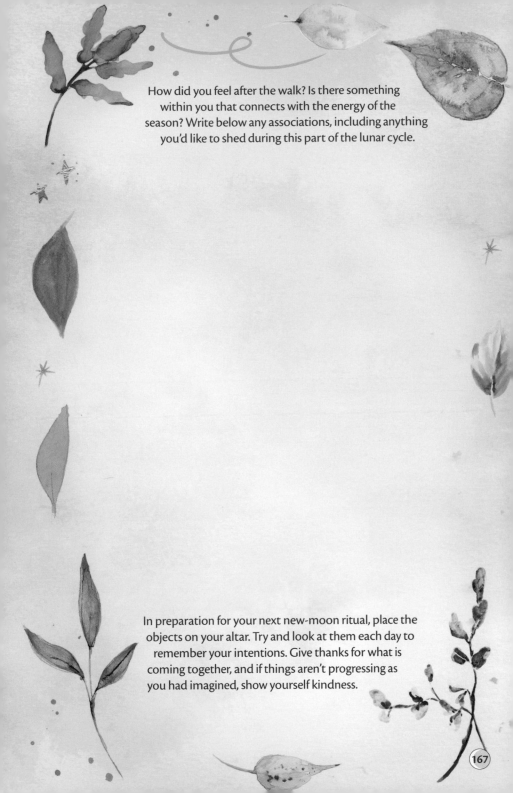

How did you feel after the walk? Is there something within you that connects with the energy of the season? Write below any associations, including anything you'd like to shed during this part of the lunar cycle.

In preparation for your next new-moon ritual, place the objects on your altar. Try and look at them each day to remember your intentions. Give thanks for what is coming together, and if things aren't progressing as you had imagined, show yourself kindness.

Meet Your Spirit Animal

Get a crystal you associate with loving support; if nothing stands out to you, try rose quartz. Hold it in your hand and sit quietly, feeling as your skin warms it up. If it helps, you can play meditative music to engage your senses. Take a few deep breaths, and think about what guidance you crave right now. Note that down.

Now, imagine yourself walking into a natural setting: a forest, beach, mountain, desert, wherever your mind leads. In this place, imagine meeting your spirit animal. What form does it take? Picture the energy you need to support you, and send that thought out to the creature. How does it respond? When you're ready, write down what you felt it sent you.

Now you've met your spirit animal, draw it below. If the meditation didn't bring a clear image to mind, that's all right: draw an animal you relate to strongly, or one that you've drawn in an oracle deck, or connect to a spiritual healer for a reading.

Crone Goddess

As the moon nears complete darkness, it's time to meet the last aspect of the triple goddess archetype: Hecate, the crone. She holds the wisdom of her many decades, and is seen as bearing a torch in the night. Draw yourself years from now, embodying this mysterious, insightful energy.

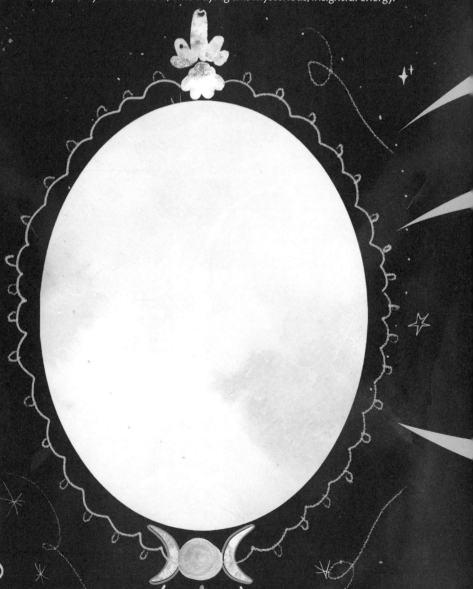

Write what you would tell your younger self, using the magic of hindsight and experience. Think deeply about what, when you reach that time of life, would strike you as most important.

It's OK Not To Feel OK

During this part of the lunar cycle, it's a time to get real with your feelings. It's common to react to uncomfortable emotions by trying to escape them, but you don't have to. Instead, spend some time completing each of the sentences below, recording any anxieties, resentments or regrets. You aren't required to feel happy all the time; you can accept all of yourself.

It's OK . . .

It's OK . . .

It's OK . . .

It's OK . . .

Inner Knowing

As the moon nears the end of its cycle, you can use affirmations of trust to prepare you for the next new moon. Recite throughout the day these statements, tapping into your flowing subconscious energy:

Everything is as it should be.

I accept with grace where I am right now, and what I have learned.

I choose to see both the light and the dark as parts of me that make me whole.

I open up to the new possibilities before me.

Below, create your own closing affirmations.

A Serene Scene

As the lunar cycle closes, ready to begin anew, it's important to feel restored. Draw a view you'd like to escape to, one that creates a sense of calm. Think of it as a scene of perfect beauty you can visit whenever you want.

Acknowledgements

A big thankyou to my parents Karen and Peter, whose endless love and support have given me the confidence to be creative in my work and life. To my boyfriend Will for helping me through my fearful moments. Thanks to my brothers, family and favourite pooches Sasha and Mango. To my amazing studio family Nina, Jade, Suzie and Ellie for their amazing energy and support. To all my friends whose love has helped me with this book, even if they may not know it!

A massive thanks to the Leaping Hare team for all their hard work and belief in the book! Monica for scouting and helping me find my way, Elizabeth for all your enthusiasm and hard work. Anna, James, Hanri, Jo, Tom and David for pulling it all together and making it look so beautiful.